There is Nothing Much More Than
the Virus
That Wears a Crown!

它不就是
戴着皇冠的病毒吗?

Edited by Yi Huang, Meiyuk Joanna Chan

Editors in Chief: Yi Huang   Weili Wu

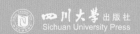
四川大学 出版社
Sichuan University Press

项目策划：张 晶 刘 畅
责任编辑：刘 畅
责任校对：于 俊
封面设计：墨创设计
责任印制：王 炜

图书在版编目（CIP）数据

它不就是戴着皇冠的病毒吗？ = There is nothing
much more than the virus that wear a crown! ：英文 /
黄颐，吴薇莉原著；黄颐，陈美玉译著. — 成都：四
川大学出版社，2020.4
ISBN 978-7-5614-7822-6

Ⅰ．①它… Ⅱ．①黄… ②吴… ③陈… Ⅲ．①日冕形
病毒-病毒病-肺炎-心理疏导-儿童读物-英文 Ⅳ.
① R395.6-49

中国版本图书馆 CIP 数据核字（2020）第 070894 号

书　名	它不就是戴着皇冠的病毒吗？
	TA BU JIUSHI DAIZHE HUANGGUAN DE BINGDU MA?
原　著	黄 颐 吴薇莉
译　著	黄 颐 陈美玉
出　版	四川大学出版社
地　址	成都市一环路南一段 24 号（610065）
发　行	四川大学出版社
书　号	ISBN 978-7-5614-7822-6
印前制作	墨创文化
印　刷	四川盛图彩色印刷有限公司
成品尺寸	170 mm×240 mm
印　张	3.5
字　数	86 千字
版　次	2020 年 6 月第 1 版
印　次	2020 年 6 月第 1 次印刷
定　价	32.00 元

◆ 读者邮购本书，请与本社发行科联系。
　电话：(028)85408408/(028)85401670/
　(028)86408023　邮政编码：610065
◆ 本社图书如有印装质量问题，请寄回出版社调换。
◆ 网址：http://press.scu.edu.cn

四川大学出版社
微信公众号

There is Nothing Much More Than the Virus That Wears a Crown!

它不就是戴着皇冠的病毒吗?

Edited by Yi Huang, Meiyuk Joanna Chan

Editors in Chief: Yi Huang   Weili Wu

Edited by

Yi Huang
Mental Health Center
West China Hospital
Sichuan University
Chengdu
P. R. China

Meiyuk Joanna. Chan
Hong Kong-Sichuan Trinity
Medical Rehabilitation Center
Hong Kong
P. R. China

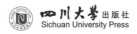

四川大学 出版社
Sichuan University Press

Editorial Team

Chief Supervisors

Tao Li   Wei Zhang

Chief Editors

Yi Huang   Weili Wu

Associate Editors

Meiyuk   Joanna Chan   Zonglin
Liu Jia Cai

Editors

Mingjing Gu   Xiaoyun Lan   Zonglin Liu
Meiyuk Joanna Chan   Linhua Wu
Tao Yang   Yan Zhou   Ya Luo   Shihong
Zhong Huici Xu   Li Yin   Qinglan Tao
Qian Xia   Xuehua Huang   Lijin Jiang

Illustrators

Ying Ma   Weicheng Wang   Wen Li
Ziqian Li   Jian Chen   Jiaxin Yu
Xiangnan Gao   Yunxiao Huang
Huaxiao Hui   Yue Qin   Jinyu Tan

Illustration Supervisors

Lili Wang   Liang Xu

Academic Secretary

Tianqi Zhang

Translation Team

Li Yin
Mental Health Center
West China Hospital
Sichuan University
P.R.China

Sugai Liang
Mental Health Center
West China Hospital
Sichuan University
P.R.China

Yan Huang
Mental Health Center
West China Hospital
Sichuan University
P.R.China

Xinwei Wang
Crestwood Preparatory
College
Toronto
Canada

Danfeng Yuan
Mental Health Center
West China Hospital
Sichuan University
P.R.China

We dedicate this book to our young overseas readers and users of this work, with our sincere hope that the strategies and experiences that we have had in China may be helpful to alleviate their emotional distress and trauma that might have brought by the virus that wears a crown (COVID 19).

About the Authors

Yi Huang MD. Professor of Psychiatry. She is a Child Psychiatrist in Mental Health Center, West China Hospital Sichuan University, and has been working there since 1995. She is currently working as vice Chairperson of the Group of Adolescent emotional and behavioral Disorder, Behavioral Medicine Branch of Chinese Medical Association; vice Chairperson of the Special work committee of Child Psychiatry, Psychiatry Branch of Chinese Medical Doctor Association and vice Chairperson of the Special Committee for Prevention and Treatment of Neurodevelopmental Disorders of China Maternal and Child Health Care Association.

Dr. Meiyuk Joanna Chan is a graduate of Michigan States University with a Bachelor degree in Art (Music Therapy). She is also an American Board Certified Music Therapist (MT-BC). She has also received her Master degree from the University of South Australia in Social Science (Counselling) and Doctorate in Education from Durham University. She has been an active clinician working with individuals with diverse needs including children with developmental issues and in the field of mental health. She became the Visiting Scholar in the Mental Health Center of the West China Hospital Sichuan University from 2009-2011 and the CTO of the Education Department of the Wuhou District in Chengdu 2012-2015. Dr. Chan has been the Chief Technology Officer of the Hong Kong-Sichuan Medical Rehabilitaion Center since 2015. Dr. Chan has over 12 major publications in the past 20 years. Owing to her substantial contributions to her profession, Dr. Chan was awarded as a Top Outstanding Young Persons in the year of 2008.

Abstract

While the 2019-nCoV epidemic in China has been brought under initial control, the epidemic has started to spread rapidly in a world-wide scale which brings global attention. In order to help children to learn more about how the outbreak might have affected them as well as their families and the proper way to deal with it, we have invited all the local leading specialists in the filed of child and adolescent psychiatry and psychology to contribute in this book.

This book contains four chapters, which are written for four different kinds of children facing different situations. The first chapter is mainly for children who are infected with the 2019-nCoV and need to be quarantined in the hospital. Chapter 2 is for children whose parents and relatives have been diagnosed with the 2019-nCoV. Chapter 3 is for the healthy children who need to be staying and learning at home (some of the answers are for children who have been diagnosed with mood disorders). Chapter 4 is for children whose parents are working in the front-line (e.g. doctors, nurses, polices). .

This unique book is aimed to serve children and adolescent aged from 6 to 15. We use Q&As to address some possible psychological problems of children in order to help them to understand difficult concepts easily. In addition, we invite young artists to illustrate the psychological intervention techniques in a way that children can understand and like. The aim of this unique book is to educate our little audiences the proper ways to deal with the possible psychological problems during the outbreak in an interesting way. By reading the book together, parents will know how to talk about the outbreak to their children.

This unique e-book has been viewed over 17,000 times only in three days of time in China. From the reviews, we know that this book has been a useful tool to educate children to understand more about the epidemic and its relationship to their families as well as to introduce some scientific coping strategies they could have employed when they are having difficult times emotionally and psychologically. We know that children's mental health is as vital as their physical health!

Preface

   A world-wide outbreak of a novel coronavirus has begun at the end of 2019. In only three months of time, WHO described it as a pandemic on March 12, 2020. Date back to January 30, 2020, the Emergency Committee of WHO announced that 2019-nCoV epidemic constituted a Public Health Emergency of International Concern (PHEIC). More than 30 provinces and municipalities in China were announced to be in the first level of the major public health emergencies status. Among the emergency strategic plan, psychological aid is considered to be an essential component.

   Everyone has a need to respond to stress including children and adolescents who are still in their developmental stages. In crisis like this, we care so much about our youngsters. How are they going to understand what is happening around them? How is the disease being treated? How do they know when their negative feelings such as worry and fear set in and the ways they can deal with them? What positive things they can do in dealing with those negative feelings? Answers are to be found in this book.We believe that most of our young audiences will find the suggestions in this book useful and being resilient in this critical period.

This unique book is aimed to serve young readers aged from 6 to 15. We use Q&As to address some possible psychological problems of children in order to help them to understand difficult psychological concepts easily. In addition, we invite young artists to illustrate the psychological intervention techniques in a way that even young children can understand and like. Another aim of this book is to educate our young audiences the proper ways to cope with the possible psychological problems during the outbreak in an interesting way. By reading the book together, parents will also know how to talk about the outbreak to their children and help them deal with their reactions.

Yi Huang

Meiyuk Joanna. Chan

Table of Contents

Chapter 1

When my life is threatened by the novel coronavirus

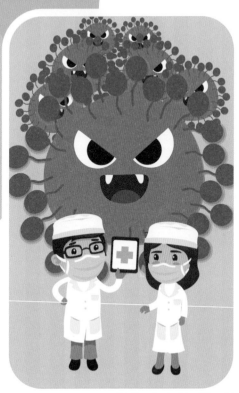

What is the novel coronavirus?

● Illustrated by Wen Li

This virus is so small that we can't see it with our eyes. It looks like a crown through a microscope, so it is named coronavirus. As it is a new coronavirus discovered by scientists, it is called novel coronavirus. It can be transmitted through sneeze, cough, and close contact. Once infected with this virus, some people may have fever and cold in the early stage. Then they will have breathing difficulties such as chest discomfort and tightness in breathing. Doctors call it pneumonia and people might die from it.

How does the novel coronavirus attack human beings? Will I die if I got attacked?

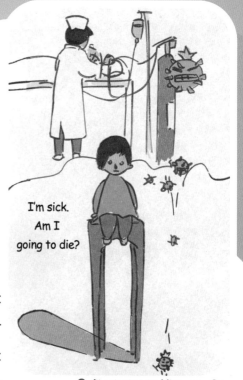

I'm sick. Am I going to die?

● Illustrated by Xiangnan Gao

Virus attack us in a sneaky way. It usually goes from one person to another through our saliva or close contact without us knowing it. It messes up our lungs and when our body fights back, we usually cough and have a fever. It is an awful thing to be sick. Most of the people who got attacked will not die from it but only a few of them who are weaker will develop into a more serious situation and die. So make sure you listen to the doctors' advice, have enough sleep and eat healthy food. With proper medication, you will get well soon.

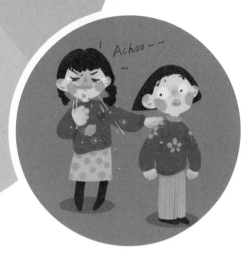

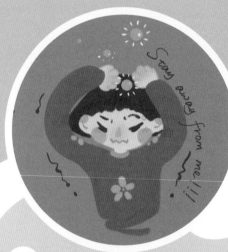

● Illustrated by Yunxiao Huang

Why can't I play outside when I am sick?

A3

Because you need to stay in the hospital to battle with the virus in order to win. In addition, there are still virus in your body and others might get sick easily if they get close to you. You really can't go out now. When the virus in your body is wiped out completely with the treatment, doctors will tell you the best time to leave the house and play outside!

Q4

What? It sounds very scary to me but the doctor doesn't say that I have virus in my body. Why can't I play outside?

People in close contact with you are attacked by the virus and the virus may have hidden in your body. The virus is very cunning and it can hide in the human body for up to more than ten or even twenty more days. It likes to play hide-and-seek with doctors so you may not feel sick now. Since the virus could sneak quietly from your body to others' when you have close contact with them, it's smart for you to wait for at least 14 days before you go out and play with your buddies again.

Q5

I don't want to wear a mask. It makes me feel very uncomfortable, what should I do ?

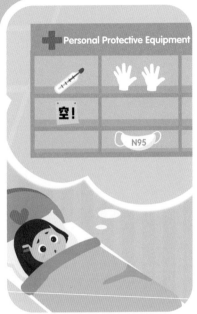

● Illustrated by Wen Li

A5

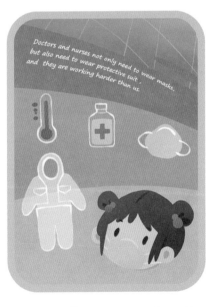

Doctors and nurses not only need to wear masks, but also need to wear protective suit , and they are working harder than us.

● Illustrated by Jiaxin Yu

Do you know how people got virus from others when they talk? The virus fly on droplets like taking an airplane from one person to another. If you wear a mask, it helps to stop it from running between you and others. I strongly encourage you to try to put on a mask as it helps to protect you and others. However, if wearing a mask really makes you feel uncomfortable, you need to keep a distance from others and use your own germ pocket (or elbows) when you sneeze.

Q6

Why am I suffering from the "new pneumonia" but not other kids? What have I done wrong?

A6

Kid, you have done nothing wrong. Just that the new coronavirus has no brain and it doesn't know where to go. Everyone has a chance to meet with it. So just do whatever the doctors ask you to and you will have a speedy recovery.

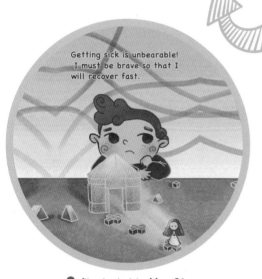

Getting sick is unbearable! I must be brave so that I will recover fast.

● Illustrated by Yue Qin

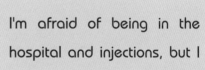

Q7

I'm afraid of being in the hospital and injections, but I have to, what should I do?

A7

Many people do not like getting injections in the hospital. Being sick is really awful but the health care workers will be there to help you fight the virus. Your family will always be with you as well. Think about how you came through when you had your last injection and the most scary thing had never happened. Talk to your parents and even the nurse who gives the injections about how you can overcome your fear. After the injection, remember to celebrate with your family for your bravery act.

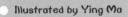
Illustrated by Ying Ma

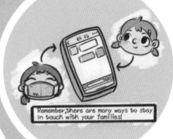

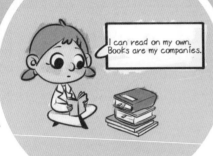

Q8

It makes me feel horrible of being alone in the house during the illness, what should I do?

It's really frustrating for you to be alone but there are many ways to help you to get through this hard time. First of all, you can always think about what you can do after you get well and get out of the hospital. Tell yourself that this discomfort and fearful feelings will only last for a short while. Secondly, you can chat with your family, classmates, and friends via different kinds of social media like Facebook, Twitter, Instagram and many others. Tell them how you feel now, and you may find a way to overcome your fear and loneliness. Finally, if you like to draw and write, you can write down what you see, hear, think about everyday, and draw them down. Listening to favorite music, and reading favorite books are also very helpful. Try out different ways and you can surely find a way to beat your fear and loneliness.

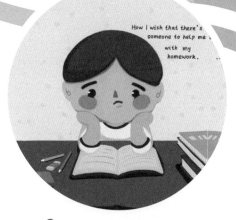

Q9

How can I keep up with my school work and classmates if I am in hospital for so long?

● Illustrated by Huaxiao Hui

Yes, learning and going to school is an important part in your life. But what you are now is a warrior who is battling with the virus with crown. In order to win, you need to be stronger than the virus and resting helps a lot. If you are worried about homework, you can tell your parents or talk to your teacher. But you know what? Schools close down now in most part of the world so that everyone can direct their attention to fight against the virus. So don't worry and you will recover very soon.

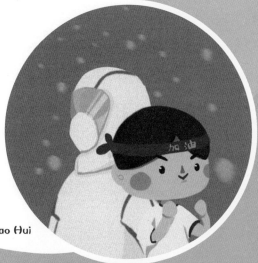

● Illustrated by Huaxiao Hui

Q10

What else do I have to pay attention to during the quarantine?

A10

Please follow what the doctors and nurses have told you to do and take good care of yourself.

If you are not sure about anything, be sure to ask your health care providers. Remember, when you're dealing with an illness, the health care providers are always your strongest support. Both parents and teachers are willing to help you and will always be with you. Therefore, talk with them if you have questions.

Chapter 2

When my family member is
"attacked" by the novel coronavirus

My parent told me that he/she is sick and cannot come back home for a while. Why my parent just cannot be home when got sick?

A1

You seem worry when you know your parent cannot come back home when he/she got sick. Don't be afraid! The reason of parent not being able to come home is because he/she "attacked" by the virus with a crown and is fighting

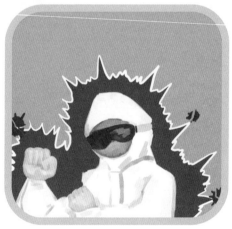

● Illustrated by Ziqian Li

against the virus in the hospital. If your parent is home now, you might get infected. Your parent loves you and wants to protect you from being "attacked"! Believe me, with the help of the doctors and nurses, your parent will be fine and home soon. Maybe you want to ask him/her to share the story of battling the virus then?

After my family member was diagnosed with the new coronavirus, I feel very lonely and cannot help but cry. I feel nervous all day long and even cannot sleep well. What's wrong with me and what should I do?

● Illustrated by Ying Ma

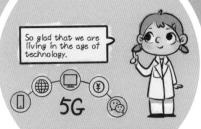

So glad that we are living in the age of technology.

5G

You feel lonely and upset when your family is not home because you are not ready to separate with them and don't know what to do. Actually, your friends will have the same feeling as you when they need to separate with their families. You might feel much better if you could call your family or video chat with them. You might also ring up other family members and friends if you want to. Besides, you can do some exercises, listen to the music, do handicrafts, or draw pictures at home which might help you to feel more relaxed. Last but not least, you can also try to think about things that make you feel happy or take some deep breaths before you go to bed. Good night and have a sweet dream!

My family members were diagnosed with the new coronavirus and I am having a self-quarantine as well. I feel so anxious every time I cough or sneeze. Am I being infected? What should I do?

Please tell yourself that it is perfectly normal whenever you feel anxious and worry

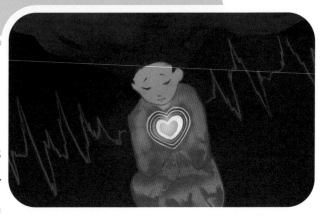

about your health. Try to calm down. Maybe you can share your feelings and thoughts with your families and friends and see what they have to say to you. There is no need to worry too much. What you have to do in order to stay healthy is to take temperatures everyday, wash your hands and wear the masks properly. Besides, there are three suggestions that may be helpful to you. First, take deep breaths frequently to release the tension. Second, you can watch some positive or funny movies, TV shows or cartoons to distract yourself. Third, watch the news on the TV or phone on a regular basis.

Q4

After my family member was diagnosed with the novel coronavirus, I begin to worry that there is virus everywhere and I am afraid to touch anything at home. It only makes me feel better after washing my hands. What happened to me?

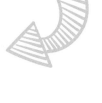

A4

It is absolutely normal to feel nervous to your surrounding and think that there is virus on the household goods at this time. However, worry of what will happen doesn't mean that it really happens. We should look for evidence to prove it. Anyway, it is a good habit to wash hands after touching something unclean. If you still feel unsafe after washing hands frequently (more than 10 times), be sure to tell your parents or adults.

Q5

Our neighbors appear to be afraid of us as if we are the virus carriers. What could I do?

A5

Honestly, we are not sure if there is virus in any of our bodies. That is why we should minimize our contact with others. It will help you to feel better by thinking that our neighbors are trying to keep us safe for keeping a reasonable distance with us, right?

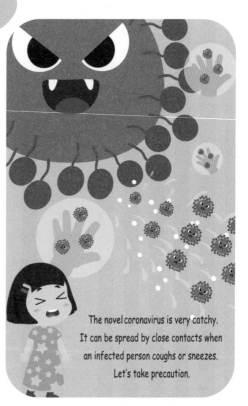

The novel coronavirus is very catchy. It can be spread by close contacts when an infected person coughs or sneezes. Let's take precaution.

● Illustrated by Wen Li

My granny is recovered and returned from the hospital. I really want to get close to her as usual but I worry that I could get sick. What can I do? Can I still hug her?

Before your granny can leave the hospital, doctors have to do a lot of tests on her to see if there are any "virus buddies" left in her body. Your granny can come home only if she is cleared and with no "virus buddies" found in her blood. On the other hand, she has antibodies in her blood which help to protect her from getting the virus again. Since children can get sick easily, it is wise of you to keep a distance from your granny for a short time. Don't worry, it will not last long and you can hug each other again soon.

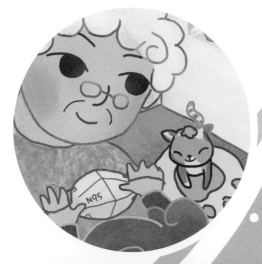

Illustrated by Yue Qin

I really don't want to separate with my family again after they come back from the hospital. I want to stay with my family all the time and it makes me very anxious If I cannot see them for a while. What happen to me?

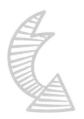

They must be very close to you, right? Maybe you can check on them and make sure that they are still there every time you feel anxious. After checking, you can tell yourself that "it's not true and there is no need to feel nervous". You can try to do this again and again and see if it works for you?

Q8

My family member is cured now. However, I cannot stop picturing them being sick. I always have bad dreams about them being sick or even dead. I feel upset and uneasy during the day. What's wrong with me?

A8

After some big things happened to us, we might have some reactions that we didn't have in the past. For example, we cannot help but keep thinking about what have happened to us even in dreams. We might not play happily with our friends as usual. We feel that way because our body is trying to tell us that it is tired and needs to rest after "fighting" with the virus. When we are charged with energy a few days later, this reaction will disappear. However, if this condition lasts for more than two weeks and begin to disturb your life or learning, don't forget to tell your parents. They will bring you for help.

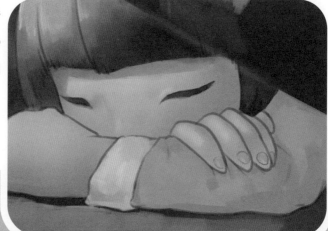

● Illustrated by Ziqian Li

My family member will never come back

again. Why did this happen to me?

Kid, I know you will be sad no matter how I answer this question. The virus
did take away your family member from you but he/she is always in your
mind, right? There are many ways to tell him/her that he/she is missed. You
can write, talk to the picture or some other ways that you want to use to
say goodbye to your loved one. Please remember that there are many
other people who you love and who love you in your life. They want you to
be happy and healthy. Whenever you are down, they will always be at
your side. Don't forget to tell an adult or someone you trust if you think you
need help. They will always be there.

Chapter 3

When I am the little warrior
at home fighting the virus

Q1

I am a junior high school student. I feel irritable and boring during the school suspension period. I always think that I am wasting time at home when we don't have to go to school. What's wrong with me?

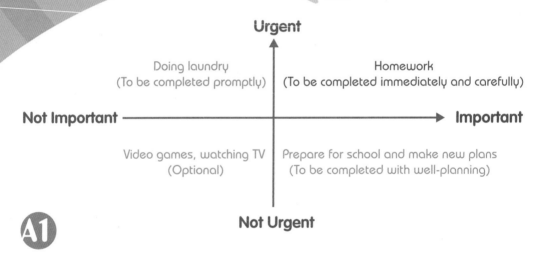

Urgent

Doing laundry
(To be completed promptly)

Homework
(To be completed immediately and carefully)

Not Important ←─────────────────────────→ Important

Video games, watching TV
(Optional)

Prepare for school and make new plans
(To be completed with well-planning)

Not Urgent

A1

I know exactly how you feel. You are just like the Monkey King who is suppressed under the Wuxing Mountain and can't move around freely. Also you have lots of the energy and you don't know where to use it up. This is a normal reaction during a disaster in young people like you. You can try to have a time-table for yourself that could help you to feel more meaningful and fulling. For example, a schedule for yourself and your family to prioritize the tasks you need to do. It helps you to get things done efficiently.

Having to stay at home all day makes me feel annoying. What should I do?

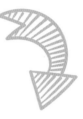

Repetitive life style does give us a sense of boring and meaningless. What we can do during this period is to try staying active by making our life interesting. For example, learn something new or experience activities that you've never done before. You might find life full of joy and surprises. You could also try to cook for yourself and your family or having fun games with them. Filming some funny movies with your parents and share them on your social media sounds exciting to me!

Q3

I have a strong will to talk to someone lately but I can't go out. I try to talk to my parents but I lose my temper or get angry easily when I think they talk too much. What should I do?

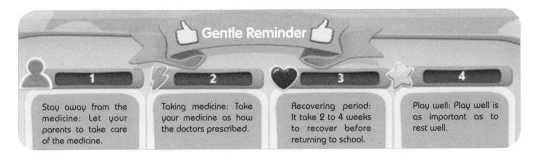

Gentle Reminder

1	2	3	4
Stay away from the medicine: Let your parents to take care of the medicine.	Taking medicine: Take your medicine as how the doctors prescribed.	Recovering period: It take 2 to 4 weeks to recover before returning to school.	Play well: Play well is as important as to rest well.

A3

I know exactly how you're feeling now. Having to spend most of the time with your parents is really not as easy. Whenever you feel that your parents are not talking in the same "channel" with you, you could try out the 4-step strategy. Don't forget that your parents need to learn how to communicate with you as well. Communication is very important.

I cannot always focus when I read as I used to. Sometimes my mind just goes blank and I can't concentrate on my study. What's wrong with me?

When people are in terrible situations like you are now facing the virus, they could have difficulty on concentration. It's a normal response. Why don't you put your book aside for a while and do something else that you enjoy like listening to music or drawing? Your study will always go better when you are relaxed.

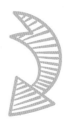

Q5

I learn from the daily news that there are people who get sick and even die from the virus everyday. This makes me so terrified. What should I do?

● Illustrated by Wen Li

A5

It is time to use your scientific mind now! First you need make sure that you are learning the news from a reliable source but not rumor. In addition, try to limit the time of watching the news. Of course, you should talk about your feelings and other horrified thoughts with your parents. Bear in mind that the virus outbreak is temporary and will be under controlled soon.

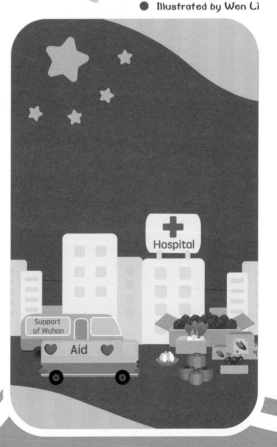

Q6

My parents keep checking messages on their mobile phones constantly these days. They get quite agitated easily and sometimes will even lose their tempers and yell at others. What's wrong with them?

A6

Well, we are all human beings and will feel bad in uncertain situations like this regardless to our ages. What they are experiencing are some normal reactions. You just learned the tricks to handle the bad feelings and now you could be their "mentor"! Tell them to pay less attention to the negative news, read the news on a regular basis, spend more time with your family, share your thoughts with each other often, and do something positive and interesting.

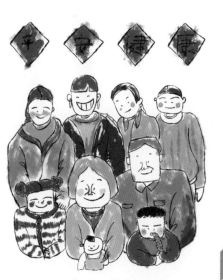

Security and Healthy

● Illustrated by Weicheng Wang

There is Nothing Much More Than the Virus That Wears a Crown!

My schooling has been suspended and I worry about myself not being able to learn well. What should I do?

You are a student who loves to learn and that is great. Whenever you worry about your learning again, tell yourself that you are not the only one but there are a lot of students who cannot go to schools now because of the virus. The government do this as to lower the chances of close contact and infection. Don't forget there are many ways to learn besides going to

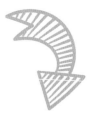

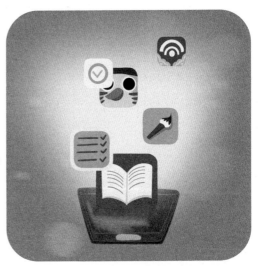

● Illustrated by Huaxiao Hui

school like home schooling and home project. Talk to your parents and teachers when you think that is necessary.

Q8

I am tested negative for the coronavirus. However, I am still worry about being infected and want to be tested again. What should I do?

Repeated checking and fear of getting sick are signs of anxiety. If you are tested negative in the coronavirus examination, trust your doctor who is a trained professional to make a scientific judgment about your condition. If you are still feeling extreme anxious about your health condition, be sure to talk to your parents or adult who you trust.

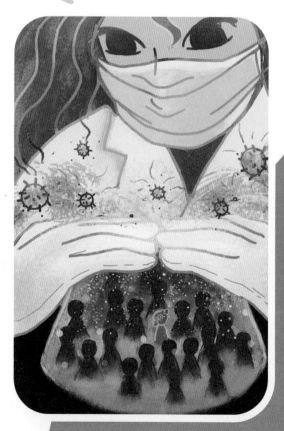

● Illustrated by Yue Qin

I am a junior high school student who is also recovering from an attack of mood disturbance. How do I keep going during this critical period at home when the virus issue is getting worse?

Here are 3 suggestions for you: (1) During this special time, pay extra and immediate attention to your feelings such as anger, sad, and peaceful. By doing this, you will be aware of your feelings that might need further help or management. (2) Trying to use the successful strategies that you have used before to manage those negative feelings that you might have. (3) If (1) and (2) do not work for you and you are still struggling with your mood problems, tell your parents and seek for medical help.

Please don't forget to read and do the following:

Four steps to manage anger

Step 1. Pause.
When we notice that we are angry, press the pause button in our brain and take a deep breath to calm ourselves down.

Step 2. Accept.
Accept the feeling of anger and try to find out why why you are angry. For example, is it because of your parents' nagging that makes you feel annoyed?

Step 3. Empathize.
Try to put yourself in his or her shoes.

Step 4. Express.
To tell your feelings and expectations honestly. For example: "When I hear your asking too much about my school work, I feel angry because I feel that you do not trust me. I just hope that everyone can be quiet and give me some spaces."

Chapter 4

When my parents
are fighting in the front-line

Q1

I heard on the news that the virus is very catchy. However, my father works in the community and my mother is a doctor who works in the hospital. They need to work everyday and sometimes they just cannot come back home. I really worry about them and what should I do?

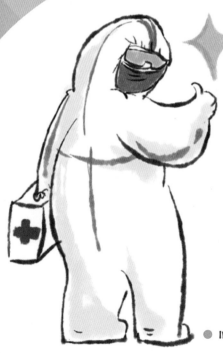

A1

I know you really love your parents and you worry about them. Guess what? I bet they know and they will protect themselves well. Relax and they will be home once they are off work!

● Illustrated by Weicheng Wang

Both of my parents work in the hospital and they tell me everyday that they need to see lots of the patients who have fever. That is why they bath for a long time when they come home and they hide in their room after that. I really miss them and want to play with them but they make me really nervous. What should I do?

It is absolutely normal to feel sad when you want to be with them so badly after they return from work but you cannot now. The reason of them not to get close to you now is because they worry as well. They don't want you to be infected if they are carrier of the virus. Please know that they love you as usual but they are just being extra careful during this specific time. Don't worry, this time will not last long then you all can get close again very soon :)

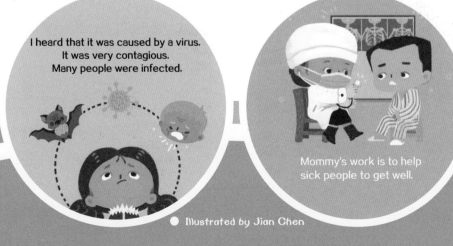

I heard that it was caused by a virus.
It was very contagious.
Many people were infected.

Mommy's work is to help sick people to get well.

Illustrated by Jian Chen

Q3

My mother is a nurse and she told me that she will be working in a "dirty team" and be away for a while. I don't want her to get "dirty" and miss her a lot. What can I do?

Since you love your mommy so much, I am sure you will miss her when she needs to be away. Besides being your mom, she is also a nurse meaning that she needs to take care of sick people. Let's think of ways to tell her that you love her when she is away. Maybe you can call or write to her? Mommy will be home very soon and you can show her your work then.

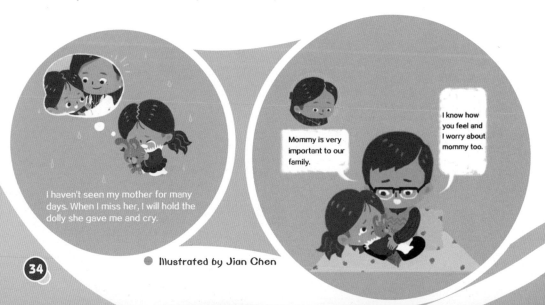

I haven't seen my mother for many days. When I miss her, I will hold the dolly she gave me and cry.

Mommy is very important to our family.

I know how you feel and I worry about mommy too.

Illustrated by Jian Chen

Q4

Daddy is a traffic police and he works on the street. I heard on the news that the virus is very infectious, this makes me very nervous. Every time I see daddy walk out the door to work, my heart pumps very fast. What happen to me and what should I do?

A4

Your heart pumps very fast because you feel very anxious and this is how your body tells you about your feeling. Don't worry, you are perfectly fine. People got infected because they did not wear masks or did not wash their hands properly after touching something with virus. Now your daddy is not only a traffic cop but an astronaut! He will be fine.

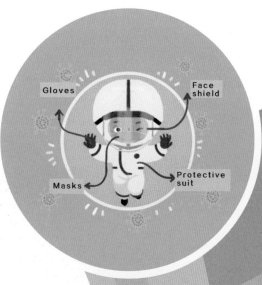

● Illustrated by Jian Chen

Q5

Mommy is a flight attendant and now she needs to stay outside for some time. She used to hug me and kiss me and I feel so depressed and cry all the time whenever I think of her.

A5

It must be very difficult for you during this time. Let's think of it this way, it might be a good time for you to grow and become more independent, right? I am sure mommy will be very proud of you being able to handle this and happy for your growth.

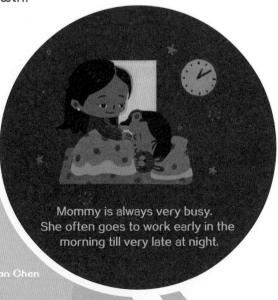

Mommy is always very busy. She often goes to work early in the morning till very late at night.

● Illustrated by Jian Chen

Q6

My parents work extra hours these days. I have no one to talk to when I feel upset or when I need help in my school work, what could I do?

A6

You feel lonely when your parents are not home and you feel frustrated when you need help. Hey, don't forget the friends that you have made at school and in the community! They can be good companions to you. If you have come across something that you do not understand at school, maybe you can ask your classmate or save it to the teachers on the next day of school?

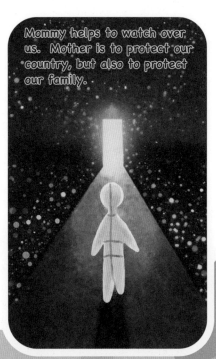

Mommy helps to watch over us. Mother is to protect our country, but also to protect our family.

● Illustrated by Yue Qin

Q7

Daddy is working closely to help the sick ones. He said I could call him if I missed him but he always not answering my calls or hung up my calls shortly. Is it because he does not love me anymore? I feel so hurt :(

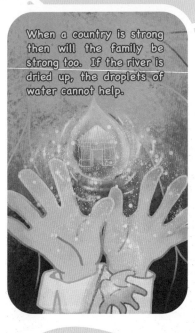

When a country is strong then will the family be strong too. If the river is dried up, the droplets of water cannot help.

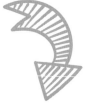

A7

Kid, can you imagine a fighter geared with armor to answer a phone call in the middle of a fight?

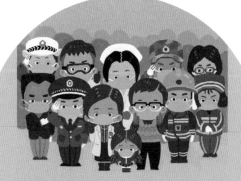

Daddy and mommy, you are my
Heroes!

Q8

If you could have had said something to your parents, what would that be?

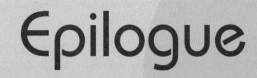

Epilogue

The sun will always
shine after the storm

Dear young friends, this is a very unusual way to start off our year. In China, we have seen many medical heroes battling with the virus. We have heard countless cheers for Wuhan and China. There were lots of touching moments happened in this special time.

After reading this book, what have you learned from it?

If you were attacked by the virus that wears a crown, you know you need to receive treatment and be isolated. In addition, wearing a mask and washing your hands frequently is very crucial.

When a loved one in your family is being attacked, you know how to protect yourself and how to deal with your bad feelings.

The more you know about the virus that wears the crown (COVID-19), the better you can respond to the epidemic and stay positive and healthy in this critical period.

You know how significant your parents are who work in the front-line fighting against the virus like warriors. You also know that how to act as a responsible citizen in a war time like this, for example taking good care of yourself and know ways to stop virus from spreading.

Dear young friends, we hope that you will learn something from this very special and unusual experience. Be respectful to the nature, enjoy your life, be thankful and grateful to others, be faithful and responsible. There will be countless challenges throughout your entire life. So be prepared and trained up for them so that you will become a better and stronger person everyday.